The Antarctic Diet

Dudo Erny

The Antarctic Diet

A Different Way to Lose Weight

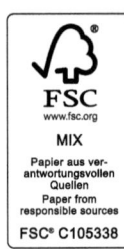

Bibliographic Information of the Deutsche Nationalbibliothek:
The German National Library has registered this publication
in the German National Bibliography; detailed bibliographic
information can be found on the Internet at http://dnb.dnb.de.

© 2014 Dudo Erny
Typesetting, cover design, production and publishing house:
BoD – Books on Demand

ISBN: 978-3-7357-0296-8

Table of Contents

Preface	7
The Antarctic	8
James Cook	11
Roald Amundsen	12
Robert Scott	16
Reinhold Messner, Arved Fuchs	21
Evelyne Binsack	23
The Greenland Expedition	26
James Cracknell, Ben Fogle	28
Cecilie Skog	30
Parker Liautaud	31
The Antarctic Plateau	32
Body Temperature	35
Diet	44
Excess Weight	51
Weight Loss through Cold and Altitude	60
Weight Loss through Change in Diet	68
Freewill	80
Closing	84

Preface

When I was 26 years old I had to engage in military service – the scale showed 65 kg, and that at a height of 187 cm. The length of my body remained the same, but the kilos began to add up over the years. When I finally gave away my tennis racquet following two knee surgeries, and was exercising much less, my weight rose to 91 kg, which was very unusual for me. Since things could not carry on in the same vein, I resolved to lose weight. I began reading diet books, but they only confused me. One book praised the healing powers of fasting, while another warned against fasting. Sometimes fat was the enemy, then it was carbohydrates. One book banned various foods, while another warned against depriving oneself of your favorite foods. Furthermore, many guides on losing weight are simply cookbooks and I am not a cook. I do not enjoy cooking and enjoy doing dishes even less. As none of the diet books spoke to me, I decided to write my own guide and that is precisely what you are holding in your hands right now.

In the first part of the book I write about Antarctica and a few expeditions that took place there. In the second part you will find information on diet and weight loss.

The book will discuss various methods of weight loss. Whether or not you apply them in your own life is up to you. The author cannot be held liable for any personal injury or injury to property or other assets.

The Antarctic

Earth revolves around its axis. The piercing points of this axis of rotation are the North Pole and the South Pole. The region around the North Pole is called the Arctic, while that around the South Pole is the Antarctic. (Experts refer to the entire southern region as **Antarctic** and the actual continent as **Antarctica**. That is much too complicated for laypeople, so I will simply use the term Antarctic in this book.) Many people have trouble differentiating between the Arctic and the Antarctic. The Arctic is frozen sea water that is surrounded by continents. Near the North Pole, the sea is about 4 km deep. The most well-known animal of the Arctic is the polar bear. The Antarctic is located at the other end of the Earth's axis. The approximately 13 million km^2 large continent is surrounded by pack ice and sea. During the six months of summer, the pack ice covers an area of about 2.5 million km^2, while during winter in this southern region, it can grow to span an area of 22 million km^2. The Antarctic is surrounded by different shelves of ice, the greatest of which is the Ross Ice Shelf at around 530,000 km^2. The Antarctic is the coldest, driest, stormiest, most inaccessible of all continents and is also the most hostile to life. The interior of the Antarctic is far away from the oceans and is thus very dry. It has an annual precipitation of less than 100 mm. The temperature during a polar night is measured to be around −50°C.

The best known animal of the Antarctic is the penguin. The emperor penguin looks for breeding areas on the Antarctic continent or ice that are relatively far from the coast. The pack ice border shifts with the seasons and penguins sometimes have to waddle 80 km to reach the sea. After the eggs have been deposited, it is the males who incubate them on the ice. Temperatures can fall to −50°C and raging wind storms are common. This is when the animals gather into a close-knit herd, to prevent as little heat from escaping as possible. The males burn 160 g of fat every day. During this period, the females head to the sea, eat until their bellies can hold no more, filling up their body fat reserves, and then bring food back for their offspring in their stomachs toward the end of August and assume care of the new born chicks. Now it is the starving males who head out to the pack ice border in search of food. After four weeks they return to feed the chicks. The chicks lose their downy coat in December. Now they too head into the sea where the feeding grounds lie. From the example of the emperor penguins we can see that their method of raising offspring would not work without body fat. The constant weight gain in the sea and the fasting on the ice are simply part of life for penguins. With people we refer to it as the yo-yo effect. Although constant weight loss and gain allows emperor penguins to survive, and is the only way they can provide for their offspring, it is not recommended for humans.

The Weddell seal is warm blooded like humans, yet it spends most of its life on ice and in the cold ocean mainly around the coastal area of the Antarctic. It is only thanks to a thick layer of fat under their skin that they are able to survive the constant cold, because fat is a good insulator. Fat is also a key source of energy for the female Weddell seal and one it needs to produce milk. The milk on which they raise their young is as thick as mayonnaise and has a fat content of 35%. I can just see nutritionists on their way to the Antarctic on a mission to convince Weddell seals of the evils of high-fat milk, urging them instead to drink low-fat milk.

James Cook

Ever since ancient times, people have believed there must be a giant continent in the southern hemisphere (Terra Australis Incognita) — as a sort of counterweight to the land masses of the north. England was interested in developing these new territories and that is how James Cook came to be hired to find the unknown continent. During his second major journey (July 13, 1772 to June 30, 1775), Cook went in search of the legendary continent in the South and on January 30, 1774 he even reached the 71st parallel. Icebergs and pack ice forced him to turn around; thus he never laid eyes on the Antarctic. Naturally, it is easy to understand why the Antarctic has no native population, in contrast to the northern regions.

The greatest danger for seafarers besides their ship sinking was scurvy, an illness caused by a Vitamin C deficiency. Since sailors on the high seas lived on non-perishable foods such as zwieback, they tended to have vitamin deficiencies. After a few months at sea without fresh food, they began showing symptoms such as gum bleeding and a poor ability to heal wounds. The illness often ended in death. James Cook took sauerkraut and vats of boiled malt wort with him on his expeditions to fight off scurvy. When the ships finally reached land after years of travel, fruits and vegetables were stashed away on board and Cook had lemon juice administered to his crew.

Every time a new magical diet is presented in a magazine today that recommends living off a single food, not only will you have lost weight after a few months but you will probably begin to show signs of deficiencies. Well-balanced nutrition can be important to your survival.

Roald Amundsen

Roald Amundsen was a Norwegian explorer and leader of expeditions. He became famous for his journey through the Northwest Passage, from Greenland to Alaska. He learned the practice of sled dog mushing from the Canadian Inuits. He adopted the native population's form of clothing for his polar excursions – reindeer and seal fur were the best isolation against the cold.

Amundsen had actually wanted to go to the North Pole, but two American researchers claimed they had already been. So he changed his goal, and his travels now took him to the South Pole instead of the North Pole. He took more than 100 Greenland sled dogs with him on the ship Fram. The expedition involved a total of 18 participants. On August 9, 1910 the Fram departed the Norwegian harbor town of Kristiansand. Everyone thought they were headed to the North Pole. It was not until they reached Madeira that the team was informed of the new goal.

On January 14, 1911 the Fram hoisted its anchor into the Bay of Whales on the edge of the Antarctic. The bay borders the Ross Ice Shelf, which looks like a 60 m high barrier when viewed from the ocean. This sheet of ice floating in the sea is larger than France and is formed by glaciers from the inland ice, which come from the Antarctic Plateau moving against the flow of the sea. The Bay of Whales develops in that sheet of ice as there is an island that slows the flow of the ice mass. It also makes the barrier low enough at that point that ships can anchor.

The Bay of Whales is the closest point to the South Pole. This is where the Norwegians set up their base camp in those first weeks. During this multi-week excursion, the team deposited supplies for the next summer along the 80th, 81st and 82nd parallels and marked them well. They would need these deposits as the humans and the dogs would need large quantities of food. After all, not only did they need to reach the South Pole, but they would also need enough food for the way back, as well as enough fuel to melt the snow. Had they not made deposits, the sleds would have been so heavy the dogs would have been unable to pull them.

The creation of the deposit sites was followed by the polar winter with its polar nights, which lasted four months on the geographic parallel of Framheim. This period of darkness was spent planning and organizing the expedition and improving their equipment. The men and the dogs survived on such things as seals and penguins. The fresh meat prevented scurvy.

On October 20, 1911 Amundsen and four companions, four sleds and more than 50 dogs broke camp for the South Pole. During the sled journey the men lived on pemmican, biscuits, dried milk and chocolate. Pemmican is a foodstuff the Indians of North America were already familiar with. In its most basic form, it consists of dried meat and fat. It can also be enriched with dried fruits and other high-energy foods. Pemmican has a very large number of calories per pound, which is so important for an expedition over ice. There are no fields or forests on the way to the South Pole, only ice and snow nor are there any rivers or lakes, everything is frozen. Thus, they had to take along fuel to melt the snow, which they would then boil to get potable water.

After 28 days and a 700 km hike across the ice shelf, which

was at sea level, the Norwegians reached the glacier that led to the Antarctic Plateau. Since no one had ever seen the glacier before, it naturally had no name. Amundsen gave it the name of his benefactor, Axel Heiberg. Across the glacier, which now bore the name Axel Heiberg Glacier, they went. Crossing dangerous crevasses to reach the plateau, it took them four days. The Norwegians measured the altitude above sea level at 3,180 m. The weather at that altitude is colder than at sea level and the air is much thinner. Since they had managed the climb, they no longer needed as many dogs and so they shot 24 of them. Some of the meat was fed to the surviving dogs, the rest was eaten by the men. Today, you would have a hard time finding sponsors for an expedition that planned on shooting their dogs to reach their goal.

On December 14, 1911 Roald Amundsen, Olav Bjaaland, Helmer Hanssen, Sverre Hassel and Oscar Wisting reached the South Pole. There is some ambiguity regarding the exact date, since all time zones come together at the South Pole. You could celebrate New Years 24 times in a single day there. With a single step you would find yourself in a completely different time zone and could raise your glass of champagne for a toast. Amundsen stayed at the South Pole for four days, sending his men in different directions to obtain astronomic measurements to better determine their exact position.

Amundsen had left a small tent at the South Pole, that they could use in case of emergency. In it he left behind two letters – one to a rival, Robert Scott, and the other to the King of Norway, Haakon VII. Amundsen's tent is now under 10 to 30 m of snow (various authors disagree about the exact depth) and moving with the glacier toward the ocean. Following a 99 day and approximately 2,600 km excursion, Amundsen returned to the base station on January 26, 1912 with his men and just a small number of dogs. On January 30, the Norwegians left their station at Framheim and reached Tasmania, an island south of Australia, in their ship, *Fram*. Amundsen sent a telegram to his brother, to the Norwegian researcher Nansen and to King Haakon VII. The ship used on the expedition is now on display at the Fram Museum in Oslo, the capital of Norway.

Robert Scott

Robert Falcon Scott was a British naval officer and a polar researcher more by chance and connections than by fascination with the cold region as the Norwegian Amundsen had been. He wanted to be the first person to stand on the South Pole. In January 1911, he and his team inhabited the winter quarters in McMurdo Bay, at the other end of the Ross Ice Shelf from where Amundsen had docked. He planned to accomplish the first part of the journey using sled dogs, ponies and snowmobiles, then manage the rest by human strength with the expedition participants pulling their own sleds. Amundsen's path had been shorter, but previously unexplored. Scott's route to the pole and back was almost 2,900 km.

Like Amundsen, Scott also had to place deposits containing food and fuel for the following summer. Dogs could be easily fed seal meat as long as they were near the coast, but hay had to be brought along for the ponies, as they would not be finding gentle green fields in the Antarctic. The southernmost deposit was set up at the 79° 28' southern parallel. It was called the one-ton deposit because it contained just about as many provisions. Amundsen's southern deposit was closer to the pole by more than 200 km.

On November 1, 1911 Scott began the multi-team march to the South Pole. The teams would start one after the other, since they would be moving at different speeds. With 33 men, sled dogs, ponies and motorized sleds, it was a logistical nightmare. The motorized sleds failed after just a few days and the teams had to pull the sleds themselves. The ponies also soon proved to be unsuitable for the Antarctic.

They sank in the snow, needed a lot of food and were more sensitive to cold than the dogs. A hard-working pony still sweats, even in the cold, and that sweat can freeze at very low temperatures. A dog does not sweat through his skin, so his fur remains dry, which also makes it a good source of isolation even in extreme cold. Dogs do have a problem in heat, since they can only sweat through their tongue. Amundsen would never have dreamed of taking horses to the Antarctic. He had grown up in Norway where the winters were much harsher than in England, where Scott had spent his youth.

After 40 days on the flat Ross Ice Shelf, they reached the Beardmore Glacier. The men with the dog sleds turned around, the remaining ponies were shot and now Scott and his men pulled the sleds themselves. For the next 200 km, they pulled the sleds from sea level over the glacier to the Antarctic Plateau at an altitude of 3,000 m. The air is colder and thinner at that altitude than at the Ross Ice Shelf and so a human needs more calories. Scott had calculated each member of the team would need the following rations at the plateau: 455 g of zwieback, 340 g of pemmican, 85 g of sugar, 57 g of butter, 24 g of cocoa and 20 g of tea. That was almost 1 kg of food per man (there were no women) per day and they had to carry it with them. The quantity corresponded to about 4,500 calories a day, which was clearly not enough for that type of toiling in the cold.

They had originally planned for a group of four men to travel to the pole, the others were to turn around before reaching it. However, on January 4, Scott had selected four men instead of three to accompany him to the pole, so now there were five instead of four. This is a sign of inadequate planning, because now the rations had to be redistributed and there were other problems as well. The tent was too small for five men. It also took much longer and they had to use more fuel to melt enough snow for five members. You cannot gather wood for a fire at the plateau, there is only snow and ice.

On January 17, 1912 Scott and his men reached the South Pole, more than a month later than Amundsen. They found Amundsen's tent and his letter to King Haakon VII of Norway, which they naturally took with them. There are pictures of Scott and his men in front of the Norwegian's tent and their faces show anything but enthusiasm.

On the return journey, the rations were reduced and fuel was running short. They could not properly heat the tent, which burnt body heat, not to mention additional calories. The men became weaker and they struggled to reach the next deposits, where they came to realize that much of the fuel had evaporated. Amundsen was familiar with the problem from earlier expeditions and he had soldered his containers shut to prevent that from happening to him.

As a result of the one-sided nutrition, the first signs of scurvy began to appear. In his journal, Scott complained about Edgar Evans' weakening state. In reality, however, that was not surprising as Evans was the largest of the men, which also meant he had a higher metabolism than the others and suffered the most from the calorie deficiency. Dr. Michael Stroud, who had pulled sleds in the Antarctic himself in 1992, believes that Evans had probably lost about 15 kg by the time he reached the South Pole. As a result, he was constantly cold on the way back and grew continuously weaker. On February 17, he died of exhaustion and starvation.

One man short, Scott and his companions now pulled the sleds with an uneasy feeling, as the Antarctic summer was slowly coming to an end. It often felt as if they were pulling their sleds across desert sand, since snow changes its known properties in extreme cold. On March 16, Lawrence Oates had come to the end of his strength and sacrificed himself so the others would have better chances of survival. According to Scott's journal, he left the tent and headed off into a blizzard with the words, "I am just going outside and may be some time." He was never seen again.

Now only three members of the expedition were still alive and had to fight their way to the next deposit. On March 20, the three remaining survivors were taken by surprise by a blizzard. They put up the tent about 18 kilometers from the one-ton deposit and waited for the storm to calm, which unfortunately it did not do. On March 23, they ran out of fuel. Scott made the last entry in his journal on March 29. That is probably the day the men died in the tent.

On October 29, 1912 a group of Scott's men made their way from the base station where they had spent the winter waiting to search for the lost expedition. They found the tent with the three dead men on November 12. Robert Falcon Scott, Edward Wilson and Henry Bowers were in their sleeping bags, frozen stiff. They found Scott's journal, farewell letters and a message to the public. They also found Amundsen's letter to the King of Norway. That was the best proof that Amundsen had reached the South Pole first. The search team collapsed the tent, built a snow pyramid over it and photographed the scenery. The picture of the three men's graves was published on May 21, 1913 on the title page of The Daily Mirror. Scott's journals made him famous and for decades he was considered a hero of the nation. Tens of years went by before authors dared take a stab at his reputation and began writing about how amateurishly he had planned the expedition.

Today, the tent with the three bodies is probably covered by about 20 m of snow. The ice shelf is shifting toward the sea and the tent with the dead polar researchers will most likely reach the edge of the ocean in the year 2300. Perhaps scientists will come up with the idea of recovering Scott and his men before then and examine them for scientific purposes. Scott's story shows just how dangerous cold and a lack of food are. There are many books on Amundsen and Scott's race to reach the South Pole, some of which are more exciting than a thriller.

To give you a better idea of the distances Scott covered and the struggles he went through, you could take the following fictitious journey. Go to Berlin, buy a rope and a truck tire. Tie one end of the rope around your waist and the other around the tire. Pull the tire all the way to Nuremberg, on to Munich, Verona, Bologna until you reach Rome. Then, turn around and pull the tire back to the Berlin. Then imagine doing it at extremely low temperatures, with part of the journey at an altitude of 3,000 m. Now it is no surprise that the poor planning that went into the Scott expedition caused it to end in disaster.

Reinhold Messner, Arved Fuchs

Reinhold Messner is a mountain climber who has written many books. For his somewhat different adventure – crossing the Antarctic – he needed a partner, as traveling the ice desert alone is dangerous. Arved Fuchs had already undertaken a series of expeditions in the Arctic, so he seemed to be the perfect partner.

Doctors told Messner to put on some extra fat before his journey to prevent him from freezing and to make sure he had some energy reserves. The trip was organized by ANI (Adventure Network International) – a private Canadian organization, which has now been taken over by a much larger organization. The crossing should take them from Patriot Hills, over the South Pole to McMurdo Bay, where Scott had originally set out. From southern Chile to the start position in the Antarctic meant a 3,200 km flight in an old, rickety plane.

The Antarctic crossing began on November 13, 1989. Their intent was to reach their goal, a 2,800 km march on foot, in 92 days. The travel organization had set up two deposits in the Antarctic, otherwise the sleds would have been loaded too heavily. As for many travelers of the Antarctic, the sastrugis were a nuisance. Sastrugis are grooves and ridges etched in the snow by wind. Sometimes it was so rough, it was almost as if they were running across a plowed field.

Arved Fuchs had problems with his feet (blisters) and his conditioning. Messner was frequently forced to wait for him, which meant he froze; thus, there was a lot of tension between the two members of the expedition. This is something you should remember when jogging or walking with someone else. One of you will get bored while the other will be overwhelmed, and both of you will be unhappy.

Messner and Fuchs had planned on hiking six to seven hours a day. The rest of time would be spent setting up the tent, cooking, eating and sleeping. Storms were frequent and made it impossible to continue. When one of them had to go to the bathroom during a snow storm, he returned to the tent as a snowman. A quick trip to the bathroom is no problem at home, but can be quite a challenge in the Antarctic with the low temperatures.

At the South Pole, Messner and Fuchs loaded their sleds with 120 kg each. From the pole, they would head another 500 km or so to the plateau, then about 200 km down to the glacier at sea level, followed by another 700 km to the Ross Ice Shelf. Their rations were 5,200 calories a day. Even so, Messner's journal entry of February 4 read, "We are only skin and bones now and the cold pierces me to the bone." On February 12, 1990 they reached their goal. The expedition had cost more than a million German Marks, a currency that has been replaced by Euro. 80% of the costs had gone to the flights and the installation of the deposits. Messner and Fuchs ended up in a dispute following their expedition, since each gave a very different account of the journey.

Evelyne Binsack

Evelyne Binsack is one of very few females to hold a graduate degree in mountain guiding. In 2001 she became the first Swiss woman to reach the pinnacle of Mount Everest. In 2006 she began her expedition from Switzerland to the South Pole, using only the strength of her own muscles. She accomplished the first phase by bicycle, cycling from the Grimsel Pass in the Swiss Alps, crossing northern Spain and on to Porto, Portugal. Since Salt Lake City (USA) is on the same northern parallel as Porto, she continued her journey by bicycle from there, passing through Mexico and then on to Panama. From there she flew to Quito in Ecuador, as she did not wish to make the acquaintance of the Colombian drug cartel. Traveling by bicycle to the southern point of the South American continent, she ascended many peaks – on foot, of course – such as Cotopaxi (5,897 m) and Chimborazo (6,310 m). (Let me just pause and ask a question at this point: How many peaks of that altitude have you had the pleasure of standing on before?) The bicycle tour ended in Punta Arenas, the southern tip of Chile, and the preparations for the Antarctic expedition began. At a fitness center she built up her muscles and pulled a truck tire around town in preparation for pulling a sled. Another preparation for the Antarctic cold consisted of increasing her body weight from 60 to 75 kg, which she did not quite manage, landing at 72 kg.

Because solo expeditions in the Antarctic are extremely expensive, as well as dangerous, Mrs. Binsack joined a group of four men. The expedition is what they refer to as *"unsupported and unassisted"*, meaning with no support from outside and no food deposits along the way. A flight took her to Patriot Hills in the Antarctic and from there to the starting point at Hercules Inlet. The sled weighed 115 kg at the start, 60 kg of which was food. Freeze-dried menus, cereals, salami, chocolate, dried fruits, nuts and other high-caloric powders. 5,300 calories had been planned per day. (Tell a nutritionist you want to lose weight on salami and chocolate and he'll probably fall of his chair!)

The expedition's goal – the South Pole- was 1,180 km away. With Max Chaya, Devon McDiarmid, Hans Foss and Adrian Hayes, off she went into the cold. The strong wind and the sastrugis made it difficult for them to advance and they burned calories. Furthermore, the group had to climb the plateau. When the sun shone and the Bunsen burners were going, the tent was not as cold as when the sky was overcast. According to the entries in her journal, she had lost about 8 kg by her 23rd day. Another entry in her journal read, "We have all lost more weight than we like." On the 34th day she wrote the following about Max: "The strain has sapped his strength. He is only skin and bones." On the 41st day she estimated she had lost about 12 kg, which was basically the entire amount of fat she put on for the journey. On December 29, 2007 the haggard group reached the South Pole after 47 days of pulling a sled. In contrast to Amundsen and Scott, they did not have to turn around at that point and walk back to the edge of the Antarctic. Instead, they were flown out. The expedition from Switzerland to the South Pole had been a 484 day journey.

If you told someone you could lose 12 kg in 40 days while consuming 5,300 calories a day, they would probably look at you a bit dumbfoundedly. Hard physical labor in cold, thin and dry air has a rather unbelievable effect on body weight. Mrs. Binsack is the only person I have actually met who has been to the Antarctic Plateau and the South Pole. In an e-mail she explained that an untrained person would be better served to go snowshoeing in the mountains than to take off for the plateau on an unsupported expedition.

The Greenland Expedition

BBC recreated Amundsen and Scott's race to the South Pole in a six-part documentary (Blizzard: Race to the Pole was broadcast in 2006 on BBC 2). A Norwegian and British team attempted to repeat the most grueling expedition in history using almost the same equipment and foodstuffs that Amundsen and Scott had used. Since sled dogs have been banned from the Antarctic since 1994, the expedition was filmed in Greenland. The remake of the race was scheduled to take 99 days and 1,120 km would have to be covered from the start to the fictitious pole.

Following a two-week adjustment period, the teams were brought to the inland starting point at a 1,000 m altitude by plane. They were to climb a 2,000 m high glacier using parallel routes, find the symbolic "South Pole" and then return to the starting point. Food deposits had been set up along the way. The teams had to navigate the stretch using the same tools available back then. Like Scott, the British team could only use the dogs for the first 40 days, after which they had to pull their own sleds.

Similar to Amundsen and Scott, the food consisted mainly of pemmican and zwieback. Pemmican is 50% fat and a few members of the team literally had to choke it down as they could not bear the taste. Not only does it take some getting used to, its high fat content also makes it very hard to digest. Starting the 41st day, the Brits – just like Scott – had to pull their own sleds. That was hard on their bodies. They checked their weight during weekly check-ups. In contrast to Scott and Amundsen, the teams took along a scale. They saw extreme weight loss. As a result, they became weaker when pulling the sleds and became more perceptible to the cold. All anyone in the Scott group could think about was food – a result of the severe malnutrition. Dr. Mike Stroud, a polar traveler, dietician and commentator of the television documentary, pulled sleds in the Antarctic himself and burned 8,000 calories, and sometimes more, a day doing so. However, the British team only had 4,500 calories a day. The Norwegian team advanced well with the sled dogs, found the imaginary South Pole and began their return journey to the starting point. The Norwegians have already been home for two weeks by the time the Brits neared the pole. Since most of the work was done by the sled dogs, the Norwegians only lost an average of 6.5% of their body weight and mainly burned fatty tissue.

The Brits were weakened and starving from pulling the sleds. On the 91st day of filming, the producers broke off the expedition. During the health check that followed, the physicians found that the men had lost an average of 19% of their body weight. What truly surprised the experts was the high loss of muscle mass. The four members of the expedition who had stuck it out until the end had loss between 6 and 10 kg of muscle. Scott's diet was apparently unsuitable for polar expeditions. In addition to pemmican, Amundsen and his men had also eaten dog meat, which the Norwegian team replaced with beef. The purpose of a starvation diet is not to lose muscle. However, too much strain in the cold with the wrong diet produces exactly that phenomenon. If the Brits had eaten a daily portion of protein, they would have lost more fat than muscle.

James Cracknell, Ben Fogle

The *Amundsen Omega 3 South Pole Race* was held in January of 2009. Six teams participated in the race. James Cracknell and Ben Fogle were part of team QinetiQ and wrote a book about the race. The third member of their team was Ed Coats. Following a preparation phase, the teams were flown to the starting line on the Antarctic Plateau. During the first stage of the race, which was about 400 km long, the teams had to find a checkpoint and spend at least 24 hours there. From there, the second stage took them almost 400 km to the South Pole.

The sleds initially weighed 70 kg. Like the other polar travelers, these three were also faced with the perils of the Antarctic. They were exposed to the cold and wind for hours on end. To sleep they had to set up their tents, preferably somewhere with less wind and slightly less cold. There are no restaurants where you can stop and warm up on the Antarctic Plateau. Since space was so limited on the sleds, there was not much room for clean clothes and you can imagine what the men must have smelled like, traveling so long without hotels where they could shower.

The foods James, Ben and Ed had taken along did not contain enough fat and they were constantly hungry. When a polar bear kills a seal, the first thing he eats is the so-called blubber, the layer of fat under the seal's skin. Fat is an ideal source of nutrition out in the cold, whereas in a nice, warm apartment with central heating, we do not need to eat as much fat.

The members of the expedition came to be very familiar with the physiological limits of food consumption. A normal person would have a hard time consuming and digesting more than 6,000 calories a day. However, when you are burning 8,000 plus calories a day, you automatically begin to lose weight, even if you are constantly stuffing yourself full of food. The problem travelers of the Antarctic have is that they have to limit the load they put on their sleds. At some point you reach a weight where the sled is so heavy, you can't get it to move.

Following almost 19 days of racing, team QinetiQ finished in second place. If you include the training phase, the participants had been in the Antarctic and on the go for almost a month. James Cracknell had lost 18 kg of body weight, while Ben Fogle and Ed Coats each lost around 13 kg. Pulling a sled is hard, physical labor that expends a lot of energy. Part of the weight loss was caused by the extreme cold. The body burns fat to maintain normal body temperature.

Cecilie Skog

Cecilie Skog (born in 1974) is a Norwegian mountain climber who has climbed the highest peak on every continent. Together with the American Ryan Waters, she crossed the Antarctic by ski. They did not have sails or other tools at their disposal. Any power was provided by their own muscle. The expedition started on Berkner Island on November 13, 2009 and ended approximately 1,800 km later on the Ross Ice Shelf on January 21, 2010. In contrast to Amundsen and Scott, Cecilie Skog was equipped with the latest technology in navigation, as well as satellite images. Both were picked up by airplane at the end of their trip.

The sleds weighed 135 kg at the start. 78 of it was the food for 70 days. Cecilie Skog is 1.60 meters tall. During the expedition she went from 60 kg to 45 kg. Her BMI (body mass index) sank from 23.4 to 17.6. Had she continued to lose weight at that rate, she would have weighed a mere 30 kg only 70 days later. Naturally, that is a theoretical calculation as at some point the human body breaks down and a person eventually dies.

Parker Liautaud

Nineteen-year old Parker Liautaud and his partner Doug Stoup completed a race to the South Pole in record time. As their starting point, they selected an area where the glacier flowed into the shelf ice. In December 2013, they managed a stretch of approximately 600 km in 18 days. That makes Parker Liautaud the youngest male participant to accomplish the stretch on skis. His record probably will not last long.

Liautaud complained of various troubles throughout the race. His sled weighed 82 kg at the start, which caused back pains as he had to pull it twelve hours a day. The wind was bothersome and combined with the cold presented a significant mental challenge. He even experienced so-called ***whiteouts*** when fog moved through. In whiteouts, a person loses their sense of direction and, surrounded by white, they cannot tell up from down. This makes navigation much more difficult and there is a risk of losing your partner. Due to the altitude of the plateau, Liautaud suffered from shortness of breath and the symptoms of altitude sickness. At altitudes over 2,500 m above sea level, some people experience headaches, nausea, dizziness, loss of appetite and have difficulty sleeping.

Even though Liautaud ate a high calorie diet (6,000 calories a day), he lost 9 kg of body weight during the race, which was a weight loss of about 500 g per day. Just imagine how much weight he would have lost had he only consumed 3,000 calories a day. Amundsen did not complain of weight loss, since most of the work was performed by dogs and he had large food reserves at the deposits. Almost all of the members of the expedition who pulled their own sleds experienced extreme weight loss.

The Antarctic Plateau

The coastal area of the Antarctic reaches tolerable temperatures in high summer (from about December to February), with temperatures near the freezing point. Certain areas of the coast are even swamped with seagulls, penguins, seals and whales. However, if you head up to the higher, more central region of the Antarctic, you find a separate world, one of solitude and cold, where there is no life or noise. There are no forests or rivers, no streets, small towns or cities, no neighbors interrupting the silence with their lawnmowers, no screaming children or barking dogs. At times, the strong winds died down and many members of the expedition described this absolute stillness that surrounded them as surreal.

The plateau is an ice desert with very little precipitation. Since sunlight falls in a flat angle in summer, it is reflected by the snow-covered surface. As a result, it remains cold even though the sun shines 24-hours a day. A temperature of -89.2°C was measured on July 21, 1983 near the Russian station of Vostok. The research station is located at an altitude of almost 3,500 m above sea level. For a long time that temperature was considered the coldest temperature ever to have been recorded in the Antarctic. However, when the temperatures recorded by satellite *Landsat* on August 10, 2010 over the east Antarctic were analyzed, they found a temperature of -93.2°C.

Almost a third of the inner Antarctic ice is located at altitudes above 3,000 m above sea level. When standing on this desert of ice, the naked eye does not actually pick up on the difference in altitude along the surface of the ice.

The distances are simply too great and the ground is too uneven to see very far at all. The South Pole is located on that plateau, at an altitude of 2,835 m above sea level. That is almost as high as the Zugspitze, the highest mountain in Germany, with an altitude of 2,964 m above sea level. The American Amundsen-Scott research center was established near the South Pole in 1957 and is occupied year round. It is not a hotel, but a base used by researchers. Guests are considered a nuisance who interfere with their everyday research. The authors of travel guide **Antarctica** (Lonely Planet) describe how many of the station inhabitants who have to perform part of their work outside in the cold do not gain weight, even though they consume 5,000 to 6,000 calories a day. Researchers who only worked at the station for 15 weeks in summer even lost 20 kg in that short amount of time, even though they were there to work and not to lose weight.

Most people who travel to the Antarctic take a ship to the Antarctic Peninsula, which lies directly across from South America. Glaciers, mountains and animals can still be photographed there. The plateau, however, only offers snow and ice and it is extremely expensive to get there. There are flights that depart from Punta Arenas (Chile) and Cape Town (South Africa). The first problem is that the planes have to carry enough fuel for the return trip, as unlike other continents, the Antarctic does not have standard airports where a plane could fuel up. This reduces the cargo that can be taken along and makes the flight more expensive. If you plan on taking an expedition to the plateau, you should know that it will cost you the same amount as a brand new, luxury mid-class vehicle. The International Association of

Antarctica Tour Operators (IAATO) can assist you if you plan on traveling to the frigid South.

The expeditions on the Antarctic Plateau were mainly undertaken by athletic, rather than overweight people. They were often well-trained mountain climbers accustomed to surviving in the cold and thinner air. I have never once read a book or newspaper article about someone who undertook this adventurous sled-pulling simply to lose weight. If you happen to be very overweight or not well trained, you will most likely collapse your very first day out. At the very least, you should undergo a physical performance examination before even considering losing weight on the plateau. I am not aware of a single weight-loss clinic on the Antarctic Plateau or any plans to open one – even though the conditions would be perfect for getting rid of those unwanted kilos! Furthermore, the seclusion would give physicians greater control over their patients as there are no bakeries or restaurants on the ice plateau where clients could fill their bellies. And a pizza delivery service which would deliver to the Antarctic plateau? That is something I would have to see with my own eyes – it would certainly make it into the Guinness Book of World Records!

Body Temperature

A healthy person's body temperature is between 36 and 37°C and varies only slightly throughout the day; hitting a low in the morning and peaking in the afternoon. The metabolism of key organs depends on a constant temperature of 37°C. Many illnesses cause the body temperature to rise. If a child tells his mother he is sick and does not want to go to school, the first thing the mother does is check the child's forehead. If it feels warm the child can stay home. Fevers in excess of 42°C can be critical for humans and may lead to circulatory failure or even death. Protein structures change or are even destroyed at high temperatures.

If a person spends too much time out in the heat during summer, he or she runs the risk of heat stroke. Normally, the body fends off overheating by sweating. Increased body temperatures often lead to unconsciousness. If the air conditioning were to fail in a modern train in summer, many passengers would suffer circulatory problems. During the heat wave in August of 2003, many elderly and ill people throughout Europe died, as they could not prevent their body temperatures from rising. Air conditioning is not simply a luxury – it can also save lives.

When a child is born prematurely, he is placed in an incubator. The incubator regulates the temperature and humidity. The humidity has to be high in order to reduce the chill from evaporation. At room temperature, a premature baby would have poor chances of survival as he would not be able to maintain its own body temperature. Preemies do not yet have a sufficient layer of fat to protect them against cold.

When a car is left in the sun in summer, the interior heats

up fairly quickly. Depending on the temperature outside and the color of the car, a person's life could be in danger in just a few minutes. Every summer children die of overheating when parents decide not to wake a sleeping child and simply leave him in the car while they take care of a quick errand; unfortunately, that errand then takes longer than expected. Leaving a dog in the car on a hot summer day is a death sentence as well.

Humans are very sensitive to hypothermia of the internal organs and brain. When the Titanic sank, many passengers who fell into the water died of hypothermia in a very brief amount of time. During the Second World War, many German pilots were shot down and died in the English Channel, even though they were not actually injured. That is one of the main reasons death by hypothermia was tested on the prisoners of the concentration camp Dachau. The results showed that death occurred when the core temperature fell to 25 to 28°C. The internal organs and the brain need a certain temperature in order to function. When that temperature is either exceeded or falls lower, death occurs.

The human body has a built-in thermostat that maintains a constant temperature regardless of the temperature outside. If the temperature is too high, a human sweats to rid himself of excess heat. If the temperature is too low, the body reduces the blood supply to the skin and extremities. The temperature around the internal organs and brain must remain in a life-sustaining range. The body is not as concerned with frozen toes or fingers – just as long as the core temperature is sustained. Many mountain climbers have had to amputate toes. Their body set its own priorities, giving warmth to the liver, heart and brain first, which did not leave enough for the feet.

Perhaps you yourself have once shivered from cold, or have seen someone else shiver from cold – especially children. When a person stays in the water too long in summer, his body temperature becomes too low. Water extracts a lot of warmth from the human body and the body activates muscles in order to produce heat. Shivering from cold is not intentional, it is actually one of the protective mechanisms the body uses to keep it from freezing to death. When we work or shiver our muscles produce heat that the body needs to work at an optimal level.

During Stalin's reign, many of his political rivals were banned to Siberia. The first thing that comes to mind when we think of Siberia is probably the **Siberian cold**. The inland is ruled by a continental climate, with hot summers and extremely cold winters. Under Stalin, people had two fears: fear of the concentration camp and fear of the cold, as these two cost many people their lives. Stalin could have set up the concentration camps along the Black Sea, but the climate is pleasant there and the dictator was not interested in the people's well-being, but in his ability to intimidate them.

When people are forced to spend too much time outside on a cold winter day, they begin to jog back and forth and swing their arms to stay warm. It is precisely by working our muscles that we can produce heat. However, humans do not make for very effective machines. Approximately three fourths of energy is lost as heat, only a small part is pure mechanical muscle work. Our muscles not only enable us to move, they also serve as a form of internal "heater".

In a closed room filled with people, the temperature rises as each person present emits almost 100 watts of heat as part of his or her metabolic processes. If a person can no longer emit heat, since the room temperature has risen, he or she may begin to feel ill and the windows may be thrown open. Some people simply say the air is bad or stuffy, but it is not only the increased level of carbon dioxide that is causing problems, but the fact that the conditions have interfered with our thermoregulation. Since humans are continuously producing heat as a result of metabolism, that heat has to be disposed of. As a result, the temperature at which the body is comfortable is not 37°C, but 23°C when humidity levels are not very high.

Each person has a different sensitivity to heat. Let us examine the following situation: There are two people in a room. One of them is freezing while the other thinks it is too warm. Why might that be? It generally has to do with a person's physique. An underweight person will freeze more quickly. An overweight person with a thick layer of fat is well insulated and is more comfortable at lower temperatures. Basically, the situation can be summed up as follows: Skinny people freeze, fat people sweat.

You rarely see divers going into the water without a diving suit. Although we can get by without protection for shorter dives in the tropics, we generally need a suit that is suitable for certain water temperatures. Wet suits made of Neoprene will probably be between 3 to 8 mm thick, depending on the water temperature. A dry suit protects better against the cold. Just how cold you can get when diving naturally depends on the layer of fat under your skin and that varies from diver to diver.

Some architects know little about human body temperature and thermoregulation. They build restaurants with large, glass fronts, because they are modern and give off such a nice tone as the space is **flooded with light**. In summer, people feel unwell behind the hot plate glass and, since the greenhouse effect is also at work, air conditioners have to be turned on full blast. Sitting in front of large, plate glass in winter will not be comfortable either, as the body will have to emit too much heat toward the cold glass. Although the temperature in the restaurant may be high, it cannot stop the heat that is lost through this emission.

Many animals have adapted to the cold. They put on a layer of fat or grow thick fur or feathers to protect against heat loss. Humans are better suited for warmer climates, where we can protect ourselves by sweating. However, air conditioners are installed in homes and cars since cooling by sweating is not very effective in hot and humid weather. Humans protect themselves against cold through clothing and by building homes with heaters. In 1920, very few homes had central heating. Usually, only a single room was heated and the remaining rooms were cool. As a result, humans emitted more body heat into the environment and remained rather thin, since part of their food intake went to produce warmth. Today, heat loss is rather minimal. Combined with the fact that food is always available, this has led to excess weight in many people.

Almost every thriller we watch involves a dead person. The coroner comes out to examine the body and tells the police commissioner exactly how many hours ago the murder was committed. A key criterion for his or her statement is the core temperature of the corpse. Television shows never show just how the temperature is determined, which is because a coroner has to insert a special thermometer into the rectum. A living person has a temperature of 37°C. When a person dies, metabolism stops and body heat is no longer produced. The coroner can use the outside temperature, the dead person's clothing and the core temperature of the corpse to approximate the time of death. A general rule of thumb is that the temperature drops about 1 to 2°C every hour. Naturally, the time of death cannot be determined based on body temperature for corpses that have been lying around for a few days.

Napoleon set off for Moscow with 420,000 soldiers. When winter came, he and his army turned around. Only around 10,000 soldiers made it back alive. Many died of the cold. Hitler experienced a similar disaster in the Russian cold. Both war mongers underestimated the importance of a human's ability to maintain a constant body temperature. Human life is only possible within a limited temperature range. In 2010, the Sauna World Championships were held in the Finnish city of Heinola. One hundred thirty-five sauna fans from 15 countries participated. In the finals, the two rivals sat in a sauna that had been set to 110°C. After six minutes, both participants collapsed. The defending champion, Timo Kaukonen, survived, but it was too late for the Russian finalist Vladimir Ladyzhenskyi. Competitions that have a significant impact on body temperature should not be legal. A semi-marathon was held in Tel Aviv in March of 2013. The temperature early that morning was over 30°C. A 29-year old participant died of heat stroke. Twenty-four other runners ended up in the hospital, requiring treatment for heat-related problems. During extreme performance, muscles produce a lot of heat. If the body cannot rid itself of that heat, a person begins to have circulatory problems. Thus, it is better to avoid physical strain during hot weather.

The Australian Open tennis tournament is held every January in Melbourne. During the Australian summer, temperatures can rise above 40°C. Many tennis players try to bring their body temperature down using bags of ice, since sweating alone does not suffice. Every year, players collapse. Even ball boys and girls have to be carried out of the stadium. When temperatures get too high, the matches scheduled for the outdoor courts are rescheduled for the evening. The main courts are equipped with retractable roofs. These are not only closed in case of rain, but in extreme heat as well and then the air conditioning is switched on. Body temperature dictates our lives in many situations.

In January 2014, a cold streak moved through the USA. Temperatures fell to -40°C in some states. At those temperatures, the threat of freezing within minutes was very real. In the city of Lexington (Kentucky), a prisoner escaped from prison wearing only his prison uniform. Since the cold streak stretched all the way to the Deep South in the USA, Kentucky was experiencing temperatures of -20°C. The very next day, the escapee showed up at a hotel and asked the concierge to call the police and tell them it was much too cold out there in the free world. A short time later he was back in his cell enjoying the warmth.

The problem of body heat has been well known in livestock management for a long time. If temperatures in the stall are too low, part of the feed given to the animals ends up being used to produce warmth, instead of for the intended weight gain. The climate in the stall has a decisive influence on the success of the operation. There are also regulatory ordinances that govern the temperature and humidity in a stall; these may vary depending on an animal's age and weight as well. Young piglets need a higher temperature than full-grown animals.

Anyone who has ever had an aquarium knows how important water temperature is. Most aquariums are stocked with subtropic freshwater fish, which need a temperature between 22 and 28°C. If the aquarium heater fails, the fish will soon be floating belly up. Anyone with a reptile needs a terrarium. Reptiles do not have a constant body temperature like humans. They get heat from their surroundings, e.g. by lying in the sun. Animals in terrariums often die because their owners expose the reptiles to the wrong temperature or place them in a drafty area.

Not only living beings have problems with staying warm or cool. If the cooling system of a car engine fails, you will not be able to continue driving as the car would overheat and that could damage the engine. At the atomic power plant in Fukushima, the reactors experienced a nuclear meltdown when the cooling system was damaged by a tsunami. This resulted in the need for power to be saved across Japan. To that end, many decided not to turn on their air conditioners, which caused many people to end up in the hospital, requiring treatment for heat-related problems.

Most people are not even aware how dangerous cold and heat are. These terms never appear in suicide statistics. Always in first place are hanging or asphyxiation, followed by jumping, poisoning or throwing oneself in front of a train or other moving vehicle. When there is a cold streak, dozens of homeless people die because their core body temperatures drop too low. If you wish to integrate cold as a factor in your diet, remember that any extreme reductions in your body temperature can have grave results. Never over do it when it comes to cold.

Diet

Life is a chemical and a physical process. Like other animals, people consume food to convert it into energy. Food intake is what makes it possible to survive. Most animals spend a large part of their lives searching for food. Our early ancestors lived in a similar manner and were happy when they could get their hands on something edible. They ate everything they could find and anything that crossed their path. Starvation has been a recurring theme in human history. The excess of food (that governs most affluent countries today) was definitely an exception and was something only the upper classes enjoyed. There was no talk of calories or vitamins. The main focus was simply to survive.

Diet still plays a central role in our lives as well. It begins early on with a birthday cake. I do not know a single person who serves their child a tomato salad instead of a cake on his birthday. Even a wedding is celebrated with a cake. Some grooms have an inkling of unfortunate things to come when they see their betrothed joyously sling down three pieces of wedding cake. There is eating and drinking at every party. Sometimes illegal substances are consumed to lift the mood. Be different: organize a party where you only offer low-fat yogurt and crackers to eat and tap water to drink. No one will ever forget you and you might have fewer friends afterward.

"Can I buy you a drink?" is a commonly asked question. If that is followed by dinner at a restaurant and the portions are small, we tend to complain. We want full plates for our money. In every film you watch, someone is pouring himself a whiskey because he is stressed. Magazines on food and drink can be found at every news stand. Bookstores offer hundreds of cookbooks, as well as gourmet guides that rate the best restaurants. A top restaurant losing a star can mean serious financial consequences. During festivals, candies are tossed off parade floats into the crowd of spectators. A cooking show is always running on some TV channel. If friends return from a trip, they tell us all about what they ate and drank. Contacts are made and secret plans devised during business dinners. If relatives come for a visit, the table bends under all the food. If we want to say good-bye, we carry on the old tradition of sharing a drink, so we can sit soundly in our saddles. When the year comes to an end, we raise a glass of champagne in a toast and we all pledge to lose weight in the new year.

Eating is actually the intake of energy. The physical unit for energy is a joule (J) or the obsolete, but still widely used calorie. A calorie corresponds to around 4.18 J. In this book I will stick with calories, since that is the unit most of us are familiar with. Different foods have different energy contents: 1 gram of fat has 9 calories, 1 gram of pure alcohol has 7 calories, 1 gram of carbohydrate has 4 calories and 1 gram of protein has 4 calories. The World Health Organization recommends that 55% of our energy come from carbohydrates. Fats should not make up more than 30 to 35% of our diet. Finally, the protein recommendation is a 10 to 15% share of our diet.

We all require different energy quantities depending on our body weight and the work we do. Our body still needs energy, even if we are simply lying about, doing nothing. The heart pumps blood, the lungs breath, the digestive organs are hard at work, the brain is thinking and monitoring our body temperature, which needs to remain constant. The metabolic rate when the body is at rest mainly depends on a person's body weight and muscle mass. Most authors do not even mention ambient temperature. Normally, people are indoors, but outdoors in the cold, the metabolic rate rises because the body has to produce heat as well.

Our energy rate increases the moment we get up and begin to move around. Even a common stroll burns around 200 calories per hour, depending on body weight and speed. When jogging, we burn 300 to 600 calories per hour, depending on how fast we jog. Detailed tables on how many calories are burned doing various activities and sports can be found on the Internet and in a wide variety of books. Unfortunately, only very few publications mention air temperature. Some even claim temperature is irrelevant. The members of the expeditions in the Antarctic lost a lot of weight because they were exposed to the cold day and night.

In affluent countries food is always available. Refrigerators are always full and a walk through town offers a wide variety of foods. Thus, many people eat too much and are never hungry. Before we even get to the point of being hungry we have already polished off a candy bar or a hotdog. The energy density of what we eat is often too high. Most people eat too much fat and sugar. 100 grams of chocolate has about 500 calories of energy. The same amount of iceberg lettuce only provides 12 calories of energy. There are dieticians who recommend an average food energy density of 100 to 150 calories per 100 grams.

Most diet books reference the consumption of excess amounts of sugar and fat. Apparently, people who eat too much protein are rare. Nutrition tables divide food content into carbohydrates, fat and protein. A large part of the population eats too much fat and too many carbohydrates, but not enough protein. It is not easy to meet the recommended protein levels. Significant sources of protein are meat, fish, dairy and eggs. Animal protein is more valuable since its composition is more similar to that of the human body than is plant protein. Protein achieves the longest-lasting feeling of satiation.

One source of energy that should not be underestimated is alcohol. At Oktoberfest in Munich, beer is probably the primary source of energy. Most people at Oktoberfest could probably care less that 1 liter of beer provides about 400 calories of energy, they simply want to have fun. Wine drinkers do too and forget all too quickly that 1 deciliter of wine has between 60 and 90 calories. To forget that fact, they finish with a large whiskey, and now they have just consumed another 100 calories. Alcoholic beverages should be considered a foodstuff from an energy perspective. Large quantities over extended periods not only lead to excess weight, but hold the potential risk of addiction.

The German Nutrition Society recommends consuming 30 grams of fiber a day. In reality, it is hard to discern just how much we are consuming. After all, who actually adds up the contents of every single food? Fibers can be found in plant material. Since they cannot be fully digested they are a good filler. Whole grain products, fruits and vegetables contain the most fiber.

The food industry, however, is very creative in its attempts to increase sales. Their products are full of additives that make us want to eat more. In food manipulation, substitutes are used for financial reasons, in order to underbid the competition. Food chemists are constantly developing new flavors that can be advertised in all sorts of media. The giants in the food industry have enormous advertising budgets. The introduction of fat-free products did not magically eliminate obesity, but the food magicians' stockholders were certainly satisfied with the results. Artificial sweeteners were unable to reduce human mass either. In the end, the companies in the food industry are profit-oriented and their motto is: growth above all else.

Since 1972, companies have been able to obtain fructose (HFCS or high fructose corn syrup) relatively cheaply from corn. Fructose is a strong sweetener, which is why it is used in so many soft drinks and foods. Due to the intensity of the sweetness, the food industry needs less raw material and is thus able to reduce costs. If you live on processed foods, it is almost certain you are consuming too much fructose, which can lead to obesity. Since fructose is cheaper than traditional sugar, it will probably be used for a long time to come. Unfortunately, our bodies are able to turn sugar into unwanted body fat.

A perfect example of the miracles the food industry is able to perform is potato chips. A boiled potato is relatively flavorless, but potato chips are available in a wide variety of flavors. Slicing a potato and cooking it in fat is certainly not a fine art. The real cooking begins when food chemists start adding flavorings and flavor enhancers. The result? People devour great big bags of potato chips without stopping because they want more and more of those additives – just like an addict. One hundred grams of potato chips have a nutritional value of about 500 calories. Billions are earned off of potato chips today. Just as long as the company's numbers are right. Obesity? Let other companies earn money off the overweight.

Decades ago fat was branded the enemy when it came to nutrition. This was followed by the introduction of innumerable reduced-fat products into the market, but the number of overweight people did not decrease. Since these low-fat "light" products do not fill you up, many people simply eat more of them. The fat that has magically disappeared from the food is replaced with other substances that increase our energy intake and thus promote weight gain. We will continue to find these products on the shelves as long as the food industry can continue generating sales with their light products and as long as people continue believing the promises made in the advertisements.

Fast food has played an increasing role in our diets since the 1950s. We hardly have to wait for our food at all or spend much time eating it. Foods from fast food restaurants are often high-fat and if eaten exclusively, lead to obesity. A few fast food chains offer extra-large portions at a low price, which encourages some frugal folks to overeat. Morgan Spurlock filmed the movie ***Super Size Me***, which criticized McDonald's. For 30 days he only ate at McDonald's and he put on 12 kg in those 30 days. After the movie came out, the Swedish University of Linköping performed a similar experiment in which 18 test subjects had to eat more than 6,000 calories a day over the course of four weeks. The increased metabolism caused the participants to constantly feel full and greasy and to sweat. On average, they gained 10% of their starting body weight. After the study, the test subjects lost the binging weight.

In the fight against obesity, the State of New York attempted to ban oversized cups for sweetened drinks. The maximum permissible size for a beverage would have been 16 ounces, which is just under half a liter. A judge stopped the regulation right before it went into effect. It is also questionable whether such a regulation would have made the overweight thinner. After all, there was no ban on getting up and getting another drink.

Billions are spent on food advertising every year. If we lived exclusively off the foods advertised on television, we would eat lots of fat and sugar and then a few magic yogurts that are good for digestion. Commercials advertising vegetables or fruits are rather rare. Television advertising tends to target children, turning them on to sugary snacks and drinks. At the grocery store, parents end up having to fight their offspring as they toss precisely those products into the shopping cart.

Robert Scott and other Antarctic sled pullers would have loved to have fatty junk food and sugary soft drinks. They would have worked off all those extra calories through their hard work out in the cold without gaining an ounce. Unfortunately, many people eat like the Antarctic explorers, but spend their days in an air-conditioned office or a heated apartment and their only sports are the ones they watch on TV. Many of our fellow humans bear the results of that lifestyle with their increased body weight.

Excess Weight

Perhaps you have seen the Monty Python movie ***Meaning of Life***. In one scene a very fat man enters a fancy restaurant, eats his way through the menu while vomiting into a series of buckets and finally explodes when he eats a tiny mint wafer. Seriously overweight people are often the victims of jokes and ridicule. Many movies present them as unattractive idiots. Even as children they are mobbed on playgrounds and later on find jobs that do not pay as well as people of a normal weight. The advertising industry mainly books underweight models and overweight women never win any of the "Miss" anything contests.

Scientists tend to use figures to make comparisons or create categories. One example is the introduction of the BMI (Body Mass Index). BMI is calculated by taking the body weight in kg and dividing it by the height in meters squared. For a height of 1.72 m the squared number would be 2.96 m^2. A person of that height with a weight of 86 kg would have a BMI of 29 (86 divided by 2.96). The unit used for BMI is kilograms divided by square meter, but since that is confusing, this measurement can be skipped for all practical purposes. BMI is a good way to express excess weight in numbers for a large part of the population. For athletes, BMI is rather meaningless, since they have a lot of muscle mass. A few standard BMI values have been introduced. A BMI below 18.5 is referred to as underweight. A BMI between 18.5 and 24.9 is considered a normal weight range. A BMI between 25 and 29.9 is referred to as overweight. A BMI over 30 is considered obese and the probability of illness increases at that point.

Because BMI alone was not considered satisfactory, a WHR (waist-hip ratio) was also introduced. In this case, the circumference of the stomach is measured and divided by the circumference of the hips. For men, that value should be less than 1 and for women less than 0.85. A higher value means that too much fat has gathered around the stomach area, which increases the risk of circulatory illnesses. There is also a very simple indicator, which can be obtained by measuring the circumference of the stomach. A circumference greater than 94 cm for men or greater than 80 cm for women is considered an increased risk of heart disease and diabetes. At this point, it must be mentioned that people who are severely underweight are also at an increased risk of death. Today, excess weight is a common complaint among many groups of the population and is seen as a threat to public health. Being fat is not simply being unhealthy, it makes everyday activities difficult and limits the ability to live life. Many people remain thin even though they live in the same environment as those who are overweight. It seems there is a genetic disposition involved in being overweight. One could argue that only a small fraction of the population was severely overweight in the USA before the Second World War. Yet, genes do not mutate within two generations – so we must be dealing with various environmental factors that are causing excess weight.

What has changed over the past 70 years? Many countries in Europe, the USA and a few other affluent countries are currently experiencing an abundance of food. However, the composition of the food has also changed. People eat more fast food and that type of diet shows a high energy density. Most people practice a job in which they sit all day. Cars, elevators, escalators take away our need to perform physical work. Another factor that is rarely mentioned is heated apartments and air-conditioned offices. It used to be that only one room in an apartment was heated and it was cold in the others. The body has to produce more heat in a cold room, which lessens its ability to build fat reserves. Today, people spend most of their time in comfortable, artificial climates, while many eat as if they were pulling sleds in the Antarctic.

If you watch nature films you will quickly see that there are no overweight antelopes in nature nor are there lions who suffer from obesity. Severe excess weight would be a death sentence for an antelope – they would no longer be able to outrun the lions. An overweight lion would no longer be able to hunt antelope, which would cause him to lose weight until he was once again slender and fast enough to capture animals. Apparently, a regulating mechanism is still in place in nature that no longer exists among humans today. An overweight person can spend half of his income on food and become obese without the fear of being eaten by a predator.

Since our early ancestors lived in caves during the last ice age and did not have to survive in well-heated apartments, they were forced to survive on high-energy foods, such as fat, simply to produce enough body heat. This preference for high-energy foods must still be in our genes today. At the grocery store, children do not go for iceberg lettuce, they head right to the high-energy snacks. Adults prefer to eat high-caloric potato chips in front of the television than an apple and a high-energy malt beer tastes better than tap water.

In addition to the genetic disposition toward being overweight, there are also psychological mechanisms which lead to high body weight. From a physical and chemical perspective, diet is actually a consumption of energy that allows the organs to function, while generating body heat so that we can survive. Many mothers comfort or reward their children with food. Once this pattern has established itself – food makes you happy – it is retained the rest of our lives. If eating is fun and represents the most important source of pleasure in life, it is no surprise that so many people are overweight. When stress and boredom are fought with food, the number that shows up on the scale should come as no surprise either.

There are people who gulp down a stack of cheeseburgers or one piece of cake after another when they are stressed. Others fight off boredom with giant portions of food. Both of these compensation measures have a devastating impact, since excess weight generates stress and prevents mobility, which in turn, further increases the level of boredom. Since food is constantly available and does not have to be hunted or gathered, we have a constant excess of energy, which the body is forced to convert into fat. Furthermore, since overweight people sweat rather quickly, they tend to avoid physical activities in the outdoors, preferring to sit in front of the television or computer. This also means they are not far from the refrigerator and the weight problem becomes a vicious cycle.

Our ancestors heated with wood. To do so, a tree had to be felled, which required physical labor. Later, coal was promoted and it had to be carried into the apartment. Apartments never used to be heated as warmly as they are today either. When dirt-cheap oil replaced coal, central heating systems were installed in houses. This eliminated the need to haul coal and every single room could be heated. This represented the birth of the second major environmental factor besides fast food that caused humans to become overweight. Now, humans have a nice, warm climate in their apartments even during the winter months. Whereas part of our food used to go to maintaining a constant body temperature, such is no longer necessary in a warm apartment. As a result of these warm apartments, energy from oil was indirectly converted to body fat. Then when air conditioners became popular, overweight people no longer had to sweat in summer or strain their circulation, which caused even further weight gain.

It is very rare to see an obese person running a marathon. This is not only due to the fact that an overweight person has more body mass to move. Rather, the insulating layer of fat under the skin increases the temperature of the body significantly when a person runs and that increases sweat production, which in turn, strains the circulatory system. Marathon runner's body temperatures rise to 38 to 39°C. It would rise even higher for an overweight runner and could result in circulatory failure. The insulating effect of body fat makes extreme athletic performance near impossible. Not only does the excess fat have to be carried around, it also interferes with our natural heat regulation. Thus, overweight people tend to avoid physical activities and remain stuck in the fat trap.

People tend to say that more slender people have a better metabolism. Actually, what we should say is that they are better emitters of heat. Slender people do not have a thick layer of fatty tissue under their skin, which makes it easier for them to lose body heat than a person with a thick layer of fat. Since slender people require more food to generate body heat, they tend to remain thin. However, once we have accumulated a layer of insulating body fat, we are less likely to lose heat. This leads to self-defeating behavior. Because the layer of fat causes physical activity to be unpleasant, we tend to move less, causing us to gain even more weight, which causes us to avoid movement even more. Fat people do not have a better metabolism. Rather, their layer of fat makes them worse at losing heat.

The body controls the intake of energy through hunger and satiation. Many overweight people are never hungry. They have eaten something before that feeling can even set in. Many people eat lunch not because they are hungry, but because it is lunchtime and everyone else is heading off to the cafeteria. A hefty meal is then eaten, even though no hard physical work has been performed. I have watched overweight people devour huge plates of food in insane amounts of time. They never leave anything on the plate, almost as if they cannot eat enough or as if they have no sensation of being full.

Cigarette packs have labels warning against smoking. We should put a warning on the chairs in front of our televisions as well: "Sitting in front of the television can make you fat." Most fattening are the couch and the TV in a nice, warm room. If we have a full refrigerator just a few steps away, then we have the perfect station for fattening ourselves up: enough food, perfect temperature and little movement. Any pig farmer would confirm this is the best way to get animals to gain weight fast. Since a human is much more comfortable in front of the television in a well-heated apartment than outside in the cold, we remain overweight. Physical inactivity and the constant flicker of the television can also lead to insomnia, and many head to the refrigerator in the night to find something comforting and that certainly does not help them lose the extra pounds.

Today, food is always available. Furthermore, there is a clear preference for food and drinks with a high energy density. If the energy content of our food increases, so does the likelihood of becoming obese. Another problem is that fats are cheaper than fruit. Someone who wants to eat cheaply will naturally reach for high-energy foods. If we spend our free time in front of a computer, we will not be able to burn off the amounts of energy we have taken in. Before I began my studies, I rode my bicycle from the south of Switzerland all the way to Sicily. I ate spaghetti and pork cutlets every night and washed it down with red wine without gaining an ounce. The only time high-energy foods do not lead to weight gain is when we are physically active.

Decades ago, fat was branded the culprit of weight gain. Today, carbohydrates are the scapegoat for excess weight. Yet, if we eliminate fat and carbohydrates from our meals, we are only left with protein. The statement "carbohydrates make you fat" is such an over-simplification, it is actually absurd. It is the overdose of carbohydrates that makes you fat. With medication we have to make sure to take the right dosage. A medication that is helpful when taken in the right dosage, can be deadly when an overdose is taken. Our bodies need fat and carbohydrates to function properly. It is simply taking the wrong dosage that leads to excess weight.

At a restaurant, everyone receives the same portion. In

reality, the waiter should ask the guests their weights in order to calculate their metabolic rates, then ask what they had done the past few hours in order to determine their total caloric requirements. A lighter person working in an office should receive a smaller portion that a larger person performing strenuous physical labor. Since waiters do not do that, we have to estimate our own energy intake needs. When we go to a restaurant, we tend to focus on the treat instead of on a controlled energy intake. As a result, we often order meals that lead to weight gain. Usually, we do not go to restaurants by ourselves and we tend to eat more than the energy we actually need when we are with others. Inviting guests to dinner is a nice way to spend time, but over the years it causes many people to gain weight. Someone with a genetic disposition toward fat build up, but who does not have the physical power to control what they eat, will have their fat cells in high spirits by the end of such an evening. They begin the evening with salty snacks and a drink, then a bottle of wine is uncorked for dinner, which increases the energy intake considerably.

For many applicants, the dream of becoming a flight attendant dies even as they fill out the application. The airlines have size requirements for their candidates, e.g. a minimum height. While they do not provide concrete numbers for body weight, they do refer to a ***"well-kept appearance"***. The ideal weight in this case is probably somewhere around a BMI of 20 to 25. Since I have yet to meet a flight attendant with a BMI of 42, those candidates were probably sorted out early on for some reason or other. Although excess weight is not explicitly mentioned for other occupations, such as fireman or police man, an obese applicant will not perform well when it comes to the physical tests. Body weight can restrict our lives more than we like.

Many books complain of the social stigma attached to being overweight. However, they fail to mention that there are situations where a normal-weight person feels uncomfortable in the presence of a highly obese person. The seats in airplanes, the opera house or theater are pretty close together and when part of your personal space is taken up by a fat neighbor, tolerance tends to die a fairly quick death. If the thinner person feels robbed of their space, their sense of comfort is restricted and deep inside he or she will begin to develop certain negative feelings. Furthermore, if another person is too close to us, it interferes with our own ability to regulate our temperature. A human body must be able to give off the heat produced by the organs during metabolic processes. The large and warm body mass of an overweight person in our direct vicinity will disrupt our own heat emission and will trigger stress reactions. If you reduce your weight, you not only do yourself a favor, but those around you as well.

Weight Loss through Cold and Altitude

Most diet books focus first and foremost on nutrition, with just a minor note that it is important to exercise. Many books claim that physical labor will not result in significant weight loss. As the examples in the first part of this book clearly show, physical labor in the cold will definitely get rid of quite a few kilos. It simply depends on where you are and how long the physical strain lasts. The climate on the Antarctic Plateau exposes the human body to three types of strain:

- Cold. The members of the expedition were exposed to cold day and night. The warmest temperature ever measured at the South Pole is -13°C. The average temperature during the Antarctic summer is almost -30°C.
- Air pressure. The plateau lies at an altitude of about 3,000 m above sea level. The low air pressure places strain on the circulatory system and the heart.
- Dryness. The relative humidity on the plateau is very low and creates the risk of dehydration, which also stresses an organism.

In the following, I would like to show you a few options of how you can use the experiences from the Antarctic expeditions in your everyday life to lose weight. Unfortunately, there are very few regions of the world where those or similar climatic conditions exist. Since travel to the Antarctic Plateau is expensive and time consuming, the experiences of those who pulled sleds at the South Pole will have to be modified to your daily life and your surroundings. Although winters at mid-latitude are not as cold as in the Antarctic, the cold should suffice for weight loss. Overweight people avoid activity because their bodies overheat quickly and they begin to sweat. This physical warming is easier to control in cooler seasons.

The members of the Antarctic expeditions pulled heavily-loaded sleds, which is pretty hard work. Unfortunately, that specific activity cannot be integrated into our daily routine and we will have to make a few compromises. As a result, we will not see as extreme weight losses as they did. The simplest method to lose weight is to take as long a walk as possible out in the cold. Naturally, you can also chose to go jogging or do Nordic walking. The advantage of walking is that you don't have to change your clothes and you will not sweat if you maintain a proper pace. The Eskimos do everything in their power to avoid sweating when temperatures are low, as things can get pretty uncomfortable when sweat freezes to your clothes. You can control your body heat by regulating the speed at which you walk. If you are cold, increase the pace. If you are warm, slow down.

On his expedition through the Antarctic, Amundsen dressed like an Eskimo. His focus was not on losing weight, but on reaching the South Pole. Dress too warmly and you will start to sweat after ten minutes and will no longer enjoy what you have undertaken. There is a definite art to dressing for the weather and you should still feel comfortable after an hour out in the cold. There are no rules of thumb to dressing right, because the emission of heat not only depends on clothing, but on how thick the layer of fat under our skin is. The best method is to start with shorter walks while you figure out how sensitive you are to the heat or the cold and while you determine what sort of condition you are in. If you work and your lunch break is long enough, you can use it to take a walk in the cooler seasons. Instead of consuming a fatty meal in the warm cafeteria, head out into the cold and eat an apple and a banana while you walk. Just remember the following basic rule: Eating high-energy foods in warm conditions is not good for your figure. Your body does not have to expend any energy to produce heat in a warm room. Go in search of the cold as often as you can. If you have to stand out in the cold shivering while you wait for the bus, there is no need to complain about winter, be happy that your body is burning the energy. If you want to warm up, then move about, since your muscles are not only there to get you from point A to point B, but also to function as a heater.

Our ancestors had neither heat nor warm water in their caves and they still survived. We have banned the cold from our lives. Our bodies know that cold burns energy and can be a cause of death in extreme cases, which is why it instinctively avoids it. If you set your apartment to a comfortable temperature in winter, you should remember that it means your body is burning less energy as well. We have a built-in thermostat in our body and we begin to freeze when the temperature is too low. The researchers in the Antarctic often had the same temperature in their tents as the temperature outside. Even if they were lying in a warm sleeping bag, they lost heat and steam through their breathing. That is why another recommendation is to turn down the heat in your apartment. If you feel slightly cold as you sit in front of the television, you can warm up by performing a physical activity. Get up, walk in place or move your arms. Your muscles will begin produce warmth right away.

Modern humans only experience the cold of winter for a short time. In the morning they leave their well-heated apartment, take the elevator to the underground garage, get in their car and already have the heater running. It is nice and warm at the office and in the cafeteria as well. The body is astonished and has no idea what to do with the overly generous lunch and so it stores it in the form of fat for the cold days that never come. The average citizen spends the weekend in a warm room and the only muscle that gets a real workout is the thumb he or she uses to change the channel on the remote control. At some point they get bored and go in search of something to eat to fight off the boredom. If this sounds like your life and you are overweight, you can change things. One possible step would be to turn down the heater in your car so that you actually feel a hint of winter. This forces your body to produce heat itself, which it can only do by expending the energy it gets from food. Instead of lounging around on the couch every weekend in winter, spend as much time in the cold as you can and move about so that your muscles turn your food into heat.

Every spring magazines come out with some new, magic diet that we can use to get rid of our winter fat. We would not have to go on a spring diet if we would behave properly in winter. Instead of fleeing the cold, we should use it to lose weight. When I go for walks on chilly evenings, I barely see another soul, but I do see plenty of illuminated windows and behind them are all the people sitting in front of their televisions avoiding the cold. Winter is a time of year you should begin to look at with different eyes. Instead of putting on winter fat in your nice, warm apartment, use the cold to burn fat. You can spend an evening with friends, eating and drinking in a warm apartment or you can go out into the cold and get some exercise. Instead of gaining weight, you will actually lose a few grams every evening and if you repeat the process the next winter, you will slowly begin to lose weight.

In addition to the cold, the altitude of the Antarctic Plateau also posed a challenge for members of expeditions with its location around 3,000 m above sea level. As the altitude increases, air pressure decreases, which reduces the oxygen partial pressure in the breathable air. This lack of oxygen places additional strain on the circulatory system and thus leads to weight loss. To integrate this second factor into your Antarctic diet, you will need to head to the mountains. Instead of spending your summer vacation on the ocean, where you play in the sand and hit the buffet three times a day, you could change things up and enjoy mountain country instead. If you have never vacationed in the mountains, you should know you will need a few days to acclimate. Easier walks are recommended for the first few days, after which you can switch to higher hikes. If you are very overweight, you may need to ask your doctor whether spending time at higher altitudes is safe for your health.

Many people do not like cold at all. That is understandable as it represents a mortal danger. However, the cold has a good side too, because it helps us burn excess body fat. In summer, I took cold showers to accustom myself to the cold and accepted them as an ally in my fight against obesity.

When the colder season came, I tried to spend as much time outside as possible. If I did not have time for a longer walk, I simply went out on my balcony for ten minutes and tried to build up resistance that way. Do not head into the cold when you are sweaty and do not do any exercises you are not already accustomed to, as you could end up with a kink in your back or a cold. You could integrate the following into your coldness training: instead of heading to the refrigerator to get a beer during commercial breaks, go stand on your balcony. If you want to lose body heat you have to feel the cold. If you bundle up in so many clothes that you are nice and warm, you will stave off the cold effect. At very low temperatures there is a risk of freezing, which is why you must protect your hands, ears and your face. If anything begins to hurt, you should go back inside. When a cell freezes, its structure is destroyed by ice crystals. Frostbite is possible at temperatures above freezing if the tissue cooled too much.

Do not underestimate the effect of walking. Walking is an Olympic discipline with its own rules about feet contact to the ground and knee extension. Competitions for men range from over 20 km to 50 km, while only over 20 km for women. The fastest men move at a rate of 15 km/h and women at a rate of almost 14 km/h. When you are out in the cold, you can set a pace that is comfortable for you. You will burn more at a higher pace, but your body temperature will also rise and you may be winded and start to sweat. You should never walk where it is icy or out in a snow storm. The risk of falling is much higher when streets are covered in snow and it is important that you wear sturdy shoes or wait until the streets and weather improve.

I recommended that you go out into the cold and undertake physical activity in winter. Naturally, you can do that any time of year. However, the hot summer months can pose a problem for the overweight since they do sweat fairly quickly and can collapse from the heat. During the hot season, physical activities like walking or jogging should be limited to the morning hours. On the other hand, summer does offer up the option of swimming. A trip to the mountains is the best way to escape the heat. Furthermore, the air is thinner and dryer at higher altitudes, which has a positive impact on weight loss.

Certain physical therapy centers have a cryogenic chamber. The chambers are like oversized coolers, with temperatures between -80 to -110°C. One goes into the chamber wearing only a bathing suit and stays there for three minutes, fully exposed to the cold. To protect the extremities and lungs from freezing, they wear mittens, tennis shoes, a headband and a mask over their mouth. The extreme change in temperature of more than 100°C between the changing room and the cryogenic chamber shocks the body and causes the blood to retreat into the abdomen. After three minutes the temperature of the skin is only 15°C. Anyone with health problems should undergo examination by a physician before exposing themselves to that type of cold. To write a book about the cold, it is important to have experienced a cryogenic chamber yourself and so I hazarded an attempt. The display showed -88°C before I opened the door and walked into the cold. The first few seconds I only saw the fog that formed as the warm air from the changing room condensed in the extreme cold. Soon, ice crystals began to form on my body hair. During the third minute, I began to feel pain in the parts of the body where the insulating layer of fat is thin. After the treatment I felt light and exhilarated, but unfortunately, the treatment is not exactly cheap, so I did not became a regular at the cryogenic chamber.

Do not set unrealistic goals for yourself in your plan to lose weight. Extreme weight loss is only possible on the Antarctic Plateau, where one is exposed to the cold and thin air 24 hours a day. At our latitude, a more realistic goal would be to lose 5 to 7 kg in a winter. Make your own little Antarctica. Turn the thermostat in your apartment to the lowest setting. Only heat your car as much as necessary to prevent the windows from fogging over in winter. Make a decision to spend a few hours in the cold every week. Hour-long walks are enough. Although jogging burns twice as many calories as walking in the same amount of time, you have to change your clothes to do it and the risk of injury is higher. You can choose any type of exercise you like. The main thing is to ensure your muscles generate heat.

Weight Loss through Change in Diet

The members of the Antarctic expedition lost a lot of weight on the plateau even though they had taken high-energy food with them. Had they taken along low-energy foods such as cucumbers, apples or low-fat yogurt, the sleds would have weighed almost a ton and they probably would not have been able to budge them an inch. Many people eat like the polar researchers, even though they work in warm offices. That is why in addition to spending time in the cold, a second adjustment is necessary if you want to lose weight. Eat low-energy foods that are more suitable to your lifestyle. Many diet books are simply a conglomeration of endless rules and bans on a wide variety of foods. The overweight reader tries to lose weight on such a strict diet, but tires of the torture after just a few weeks. Thus, try to put together a low-energy diet that tastes good to you. One that you could maintain the rest of your life.

There are no rivers or lakes on the Antarctic Plateau. The members of the expedition had to take their own fuel with them to melt snow as well. They quenched their thirst with water and soup, since the weight restrictions prevented them from loading up the sleds with energy drinks. If you have not just spent many hours doing hard work in the cold, then there is no reason to use high-energy drinks to quench your thirst. Sugary drinks should be considered a foodstuff. If you do not want to eliminate those types of beverages from your meals, then at least make a compromise: place a large glass of water on the table and a small glass with your favorite drink. The water serves the physiologic need for liquid, while the sweet drink is your treat.

Amundsen and Scott created deposits along the way, as they were unable to take along all of the food they needed for such a long trip. They had to be very disciplined and only eat as much as they had planned in advance each day. If they had gobbled up everything on the sled during a hunger attack, they would have been left with nothing to eat. Scott made the error of setting up deposits that were not large enough and that were too far from the South Pole, which cost everyone on his expedition their lives. Most overweight people have a different problem: the food deposits in the kitchen and refrigerator are too large. If I had a supply of pralines and chocolates in my apartment, they would disappear like snow in the sun. That is why as part of my shopping ritual, I chose Monday as my chocolate day. A single bar of chocolate is added to my shopping cart and has to last the entire week.

Losing weight can be a many-year fight against the pound. Sometimes, smaller steps help us along, even if we do not notice the impact. Many people crave hot teas or soups in winter. Our body knows many tricks for getting us to consume energy in the form of food. With hot soup the organism gets calories and heat, and both increase body weight. If you eat a salad rather than soup your body has to produce its own heat, which it can only do by converting food or fat cells into heat. If you wander through an outdoor market in the winter when it is cold and suddenly crave a cup of hot mulled wine, remember, it is just one of your body's tricks to saving energy. The mulled wine gives your body sugar, alcohol and warmth and that is precisely what that sneaky little devil uses to create body fat. You should trick him instead – order a cold glass of sparkling water.

Deciding to lose weight is a wish that is much too vague. What you actually need to do is set concrete goals, such as: I will eat one piece of fruit a day. These should be resolutions you set for your life and changes you make in your life that you can follow for many years. Most diets fail after just a few weeks because they are too complicated and they turn the overweight person's life upside down. If you resolve, e.g., to begin by ordering a glass of sparkling water with your meal when you go to a restaurant and then to follow it by a beer, that is something you can do the rest of your days. The resolution never to drink beer again often fails after a few weeks or months. We are often forced to make compromises in life. If you restrict your consumption of alcohol by quenching your thirst with water and considering beer or wine to be an accompanying treat, you will save many calories over the years. Have you ever heard of a machine where you pour wine, beer or soda into the top and it returns fat at the bottom? The human body is exactly that type of a magical machine; however, it keeps the fat, placing it on the hips, stomach and under the skin.

Think long-term. Amundsen began preparing for his polar expedition while he was still in Norway. Then, following a long journey by ship, he set up a few deposits in the Antarctic, spent the winter there in the polar night and did not head off to the South Pole until summer. He returned from that trip after 99 days of travel in the cold. Today, people do not have the time for such undertakings and that is why so many diet books promise that their method will allow you to lose weight quickly and effortlessly. Yet, their methods require you to change your entire life and the overweight person tortures himself or herself with strange shakes and exotic meals and then give up on the diet after just a few weeks. If I were to recommend an onion diet in which you were to eat a red onion for breakfast, onion soup for lunch and a steamed onion for dinner, your friends would all begin to avoid you after no more than a week and even though you would have lost weight after two weeks, you would give up on this onion-eating torture and go back to eating as you used to. Soon, you would be right back at the same weight you were before the diet.

Dividing foods into good and bad is silly, unless you are talking about poisonous mushrooms or spoiled food. While a sausage may have many calories per pound, it is also high-energy. What is damaging to body weight is the quantity. If you only eat 100 grams of sausage a day and nothing else you will certainly lose weight – and you will have just invented a new diet: losing weight with sausage! Various books and the Internet offer calorie information for all sorts of foods. Living mainly off foods with a high calorie count per 100 grams is only unproblematic if you perform hard physical labor every day. However, if your activities are sedentary, you would need to reduce the energy density of your meals. Instead of eating sausage and bread, you could introduce a third, low-energy product such as a tomato or cucumber. If that causes you to eat less sausage, you will have greater success over the long term than you would if you tried to stop eating sausage altogether.

In the Stone Age, people spent a large part of their time searching for or hunting for something edible. I hardly think they ate three meals a day as so many people do today. If they found a tree full of juicy fruits, they ate their fill of it and then moved on. No one looked at his watch to see if it was time to eat. The modern human has breakfast when he gets up in the morning, works in a cube farm, has lunch in the cafeteria, continues working and then eats again in the evening. This allocation of three meals per day may be advantageous to the working world, but it is not necessarily natural. If you prefer to eat five times a day, just make sure they are smaller portions. Unfortunately, at the cafeteria everyone is given the same amount of food and many are afraid of leaving any on their plates. They prefer to eat everything and the body then turns it into fat.

One of the most difficult things in life is to change our own behavior. Someone who has staved off frustration and boredom with food for years, will have a hard time changing, but it is possible. You can begin with a simple resolution: Comfort walking instead of comfort eating when you are frustrated. In many diet books, we read about people who get upset at work and then eat seven hamburgers at night to feel better. This increases their body weight, which makes them even more frustrated, and they eat even more to make themselves feel better. Buy some comfortable shoes and call them your frustration shoes. Every time you are frustrated, put on those shoes and head out to escape your frustration.

The chair in front of the television is pretty much the last place on Earth where you will lose weight. Millions of people spend three to four or more hours every day in front of the TV and many of them are overweight. If you spend too much time in front of the television and on the Internet, but would like to lose weight, then that is where you need to start – every device can be switched off. Sign a contract with yourself and earn your TV time with physical activity. One hour of walking in the cold will earn you two hours of

TV or Internet. You will also sleep better if you spend less time in front of a screen.

Elvis Presley gained a lot of weight during his lifetime. One of his favorite foods was a sandwich with peanut butter and banana, sometimes with a side of bacon, which made it even more energy-rich. These calorie bombs would actually be a good food for a polar researcher. But, since Elvis was not performing heavy physical work in the extreme cold, turning all those calories into muscle work and heat, his body produced fat from it. If you think you can solve your personal problems with fatty foods, Elvis' case should show you that all you are doing is creating yet another problem, that of being overweight.

People who are on diets that cause them to be hungry for extended periods often binge eat and have wild cravings that result in cleaning out the entire refrigerator. It is possible to lose weight without being hungry all the time. You may not lose weight as quickly, but it will be less painful and more successful over the long term. Many people who are overweight are never hungry. Then, when they suddenly feel hungry all of the time, they are completely overwhelmed. The Antarctic explorers also suffered from a lack of food, but there was no refrigerator filled to overflowing anywhere nearby. They were busy pulling sleds, setting up tents and melting snow just to have a drink, so they had plenty of distractions. Things are easier in the Antarctic than at home. Here we have bakeries and fast food joints, and it is hard to pass them by when our stomach is growling. In the very beginning, you could decide to only feel hungry for short periods or only on certain days. The feeling of hunger should never be so great that you lose control over what you eat.

Most people have a fairly good sense of hot and cold. They consider a certain temperature range to be comfortable based on how thick their own layer of fat is. Any deviation from that range is seen as a disruption to their well-being. Many people have a difficult time determining exactly when they feel hungry and when they feel full. An experiment was once performed in which a soup bowl was placed on a table that was secretly connected to a hose hidden under the table. As the test people ate, the soup bowls were secretly refilled using the hose, so the bowls were never empty. Most of the participants ate more than just one bowlful of soup. Most cooks in restaurants try to impress guests with large portions to keep them coming back. Someone who still has half a plate of food left may not even notice they are already full or may not notice until it is too late. After years of going to restaurants, he or she will certainly notice it no later than when the scale starts showing a strange three-digit figure. A feeling of fullness tends to set in when we eat more slowly. Food chemists have optimized their products so that we eat and eat, not noticing when we should stop. Psychologists have found out that people have a hard time putting a half-eaten bag away. Although flavor tricks and behavioral psychology have allowed the food industry to increase sales, it has also increased the population's body weight. A manager or stockholder shares in a company's profit and is not punished when millions of people are overweight. Do not buy large packages, even if they are cheaper per ounce. You will just have to spend those savings on diet books and books on how to lose weight years later.

Many diet books are simply cookbooks and everything revolves around food. The way weight loss worked on the

Antarctic Plateau is similar to a device with four control settings: food intake, work, cold, altitude above sea level and humidity. The food intake controller is limited by the weight of the sled and the other three are basically set at the limit of tolerability. Most diet books only address the food controller, promising their recipes and selected foods will allow you to lose weight effortlessly. If it is actually so easy why are millions of people still plagued with being overweight? Even in the Antarctic that excess fat is only removed through hard work in the cold and at a high altitude. What can be earned effortlessly is money as pretty pictures of ready-to-eat meals deceive people about how hard it really is to lose weight.

If you do not have time for physical activity in the cold, but spend an hour every day shopping and cooking, you should rethink your priorities. With the overweight, almost everything revolves around food. For psychological reasons, I hold it to be fundamentally wrong to occupy oneself with food all the time. That is why it is so important to make time for physical activity, instead of wasting it on shopping and cooking. If the effort involved in preparing a meal is so great that you fall onto the couch exhausted after every meal and are unable to work up the energy to undertake anything else, you should probably skip cooking a few days a week.

I would like to make a few suggestions on how to eat in a less time-consuming way, so that you can spend more time outside in the cold: peel a cucumber, cut it into thin slices and place it in a bowl with one portion of low-fat yogurt or cottage cheese. Add any seasonings you like and enjoy it with a slice of whole-grain bread. High-protein dried meat, a tomato and a slice of dark bread – that should be enough for an evening meal.

Slice up a banana or an apple and mix it with yogurt – and you already have a meal.

Many pharmacies offer shakes that contain many vitamins and minerals and can be used to replace a meal. Although it is not a good idea to live exclusively from shakes for any period of time, they could replace your dinner once a week to save time. A shake can be prepared and drunk in no time, and now you have time to take a small expedition in the cold to show those fat cells exactly who is in charge.

Stone Age people were more than likely only familiar with honey and a few fruits that tasted sweet. The industrial production of sugar from sugar beets has probably only been around for 200 years. Sugar never really played a role in the history of humans as it does today. Our early ancestors did not have to resist the temptation of cakes or sweetened drinks. Furthermore, they ate the meat of wild animals, which is not as fatty as the overbred cattle we consume. Instead of wandering through the supermarket with a calorie chart, simply stick to what people ate early on. I do not wish to impose bans on you. Rather, I would like to recommend that you adjust your diet to your particular circumstances. Sugar provides energy and was part of Robert Scott's meal plan, but his ration was too small for the strenuous work he was performing in the cold. Our sugar consumption is much too high for sitting around in the warmth.

Most physicians recommend overweight patients perform strength training to increase their muscle mass. Muscles burn more calories than body fat. If there is not a fitness center in your area, you can make do with an exercise mat, a set of weights and a stepping board. A wide variety of books and Internet sites are available where you can find information on how to exercise using these devices. Although exercising at home is not as effective as strength training at a fitness center, it is still a better way to increase your strength and burn calories than sitting in front of the television. When you come home in winter, frozen from your walk, do not make yourself a cup of hot chocolate. Instead, warm yourself up with these devices. Whenever possible, try to generate body heat using your muscles and not with hot drinks. Your fat cells may be of a different opinion, but they are precisely what you are trying to get rid of.

There are diet books that claim you cannot lose weight over the long term because your body defends its own weight. The body sets clear priorities and one of the very first things it defends is its temperature. Many Antarctic explorers found out that the body has no special regard for fat cells and breaks them down in the extreme cold to maintain its temperature. A household freezer has a recommended temperature of -18°C. On the Antarctic Plateau, it is usually colder than that and the expedition members slept in tents. When our body temperature falls too low, it places us at risk of death. That is why the internal organs and the brain guard their heat and it is our hands and feet that freeze. Our temperature regulation is pretty cruel. Our bodies would rather we get frostbite than to take away any warmth from our internal organs. It is in this fight for body heat that fat cells pull the short straw.

A few books recommend rewarding yourself with a piece of candy at the end of a diet day. From a psychological perspective I find such suggestions to be completely off the mark. We should not reward ourselves with food – that is exactly what is at the heart of many overweight people's problem – they find most of their satisfaction in food. Give yourself a different type of reward: take a day trip, go to the movies, or buy yourself a set of weights! Food should be our source of nutrition allowing the body to survive. Find a hobby that makes your happy and introduces a bit of variety into your life. Buy yourself a camera and photograph all of the towns and hills in your area. Eliminate food as the center of your life. Make it secondary to all of your other activities and interests.

In addition to diets, surgeries have begun to play an increasing role in weight loss in recent years. According to the guideline published by the German Society for Obesity, surgery is recommended for those with a BMI over 40. Such significant amounts of excess weight pose a risk to our health, but surgical interventions are not free of risk either. Depending on the type of operation and the surgeon, 0.1 to 1% of patients die from complications and complications are common in many stomach operations. If I had the choice between pulling a sled across the Antarctic Plateau and spending time on the operating table, I would definitely chose freezing. Life is full of risks. Statistics have shown that the rate of heart attacks increases during important soccer games. Skinny models die someday too. It is up to you to decide what you want to do with your life.

Every person reacts differently to diets, which is why I want to say one last thing about normal distribution. If you measure the height of 900 randomly selected people, you will come to the following conclusion: only very few people are very short or very tall. Most people have an average height. The chart displaying this measurement looks like a flat bell with a bump in the middle and sharp edges. If 900 overweight people go on the exact same diet, a few will lose 1 to 3 kg, while a few will lose 11 to 14 kg. Most participants, however, will be somewhere between these two extremes. If an acquaintance tells you that a certain diet did nothing for them, that statement is fairly meaningless, since we do not know where his results were in the normal distribution. This makes it difficult to predict how a diet will work.

If you suffer from being underweight and want to gain weight, you will need to behave in the opposite manner of a diet. Avoid cold and movement. Put on warm clothes so you never freeze. Drink warm beverages so your body does not have to produce its own heat. Turn up the heat in winter so you are warm enough. If you feel too full and have hot flashes after eating larger portions, eat multiple small and high-energy meals throughout the course of the day. These tips are naturally only for people who truly wish to gain wait. BMIs below 17.5 are considered anorexia. This book cannot heal anorexics, they need professional help.

Freewill

Many philosophers have studied the question of whether humans have freewill. To that end, Arthur Schopenhauer wrote, man "cannot will what he wills." We are usually not even aware that we are simply running genetic programs. Penguins in the Antarctic take major hurdles in stride in order to raise their young and we humans run a similar program. We are controlled by hunger, thirst and other feelings. When we are thirsty, we cannot wish the feeling away no matter what we do, and the feeling does not go away until we have drunk something. Why do dogs pull the sleds? Is it their free will? Why did Amundsen want to go to the South Pole? He probably wanted to become famous, and he succeeded. But was it his freewill that caused him to take on such efforts or was it simply a genetic program that rewards victors?

Reptiles need an external source of heat to regulate their temperature, which is why they lay in the sun. Similar behavior can be seen in people. On the first nice weekend after a long cold winter, we go for a walk and either look for a sunny table at an outdoor restaurant or a park bench in the sun. The tables and benches in the shade remain empty. This is not a voluntary behavior. Rather, it is controlled by our body's temperature regulation. Six months later, the reverse behavior sets in. On a sunny, hot summer day people look for a table in the shade at that outdoor restaurant. The benches in the park that are in the sun remain empty, while people crowd the benches in the shade. This is also controlled by our body signals, as our body knows that cold and heat are not good for our natural functions.

When people go for a walk on a cold winter day, they have usually had enough after just an hour. The body loses too much energy staying warm and begins to pester the person with a runny nose or cold fingers. In reaction, we look for a nice spot in a cafe and order a hot cup of tea, over even better, a cup of hot chocolate. Although we could order an ice cold mineral water, our body knows what is good for it and suppresses such thoughts. A hot drink helps our organism save the energy it needs to warm up a chilly body. Furthermore, hot chocolate has fat and sugar, which replaces the energy we lost out in the cold. This example shows how we are controlled by our body temperature and our energy budget, which reward us by making us feel comfortable when we are warm. At some point the cup has been drunk and we say, "Brrr, time to head back into the cold."

One mean joke could be, "An overweight person walks past a bakery." And there the joke ends, because the overweight often do not walk by; instead, they stop and buy something to eat. What about freewill in this case? It is important to know that individual cells have a will as well. Fat cells do not want to give up their fat, they want to keep it. When the cream puff in the window of the bakery catches our eye, that information is passed on to the brain and our fat cells stand up and say, "Eyes, look again – Brain, tell him he should stop – Tell him he should go in – Reward him – Mmm, that was delicious." That is basically how the fight between us and our fat cells ends. Often, our freewill gets trampled.

If you open up a telephone book or do an Internet search for a **nutritional counselor** or **nutritional counseling**, you will find innumerable entries. But, if you search the term **Freewill Counseling**, I am fairly certain you will find next to nothing.

Most people know enough about nutrition, but they lack the determination to act on that knowledge. How can we force ourselves to crave a cucumber more than chocolate? How can we force ourselves to crave the cold instead of a warm living room? As long as maintaining a constant temperature is more important to the body than our weight, we will have a hard time losing that weight. There is a saying, "Where there's a will, there's a way." A slight variation could be, "Where there is no will, there is a couch in front of a television." Since those are two of the most fattening things in our lives, it would be nice if we could buy the freewill to get up and go out in the cold. Everything in life would be so much easier if we did not get hungry, if it were not so cold outside and if cake did not taste so good.

Is it our freewill to love chocolate more than salad? We are regulated and life often does what it wants with us, without us evening noticing. As Sigmund Freud has already stated, we are not the masters of our own house. The body's metabolism generates a desire for food and drink. With that knowledge, we can do no more than outsmart our freewill. If you drink enough water every day, you will not get thirsty and you will also consume fewer calories than if you were to drink sweetened carbonated water. If you eat enough cucumbers and tomatoes, you will be less hungry than if your stomach is empty. If you crave salami or cake, then you know it is simply your fat cells having a panic attack. If you are overweight, your body already has enough reserves for you to survive for weeks. Objectively speaking, it is rather absurd that the body throws such a fit and tortures us all in an attempt to get us to eat.

Exactly what a strong will can manage, I would like to show

you using the example of Callas, the opera singer. Maria Callas was born in 1923 in New York, the child of Greek immigrants. When she emigrated back to Athens with her mother and sister at the age of 13, she was not particularly heavy. There, she was spoiled by Greek relatives with good food and gained a lot of weight. During the war she lost a lot of weight again, as food was scarce. In 1946 she returned to the USA and once more gained a lot of weight. At times, she weighed more than 100 kg at a height of 1.73. At the age of 29, she decided to lose weight. Her weight diary that she wrote during different opera performances from December of 1953 to April of 1954 is famous. She lost 28 kg in 16 months. If you look at pictures of her in the years that followed she did not return to her old weight, unlike so many others who end up at their old original weight just a few years after a diet.

What would you have answered if you had been alive in Amundsen's time and he would have posed the following question: "First, we are going to travel through the pack ice to the Antarctic in a wooden ship. There, we will build a hut and spend a few weeks setting up deposits. After that, we will spend the winter in the cold and dark, so that we can take a three-month journey to the South Pole and back the following summer. Along the way, we will shoot most of the dogs. One of us may even fall into the crevasse of a glacier or freeze to death. Do you want to come along?" I think you would have kindly turned him down. Amundsen wanted to reach the South Pole at any price and risked his life to do so, taking immense strains and stresses in stride. Most of us would have preferred to stay in a warm living room than to torture ourselves in the Antarctic.

Closing

If I were to enter a bookstore and read on the cover of a travel guide that I could hike from the Antarctic coast to the South Pole in just three days, that it would be easy and I would not freeze, that the sled would be light as a feather, that I would not encounter any sastrugis, that there would be no wind and plenty of sun, that there would be no snow storms, that the tent would erect itself, then I would laugh and place the book back on the shelf. However, many diet books also promise the stars in the sky. According to them, you will effortlessly drop those extra pounds in a very short amount of time eating delicious meals – just like that, without going hungry. The explorers in the Antarctic suffered in agony. Not to lose weight, but to reach the South Pole. The weight loss was actually an unwanted side effect.

The Antarctic Diet is not one of those magical or miracle diets. You have to work for your weight loss. The climatic conditions on the Antarctic Plateau are unique and it is the only place, perhaps with the exception of the High Alps, you will be able to lose a lot of weight in a short amount of time. At mid-latitude, with four seasons, you will naturally never see the same results. Depending on how overweight you are, you should probably spread your weight loss across multiple winters. Although you may be able to lose weight quickly on a power diet, once the diet is over, you will soon be back at your old weight. Instead of putting on winter padding, you should use that time of year to get rid of it. Temporary diets are often pointless, which is why you should set long-term goals for yourself and use winter to help you control your weight from now on.

Humans instinctively fear the cold, as it can be deadly. Once you lose those first kilos, you will begin to see winter with different eyes. An overweight person, who avoids any kind of physical exertion in summer, can do much more at temperatures around the freezing point without sweating or without fear of heat stroke. You will soon greet every cold snap, as it will mean the time has come when you can lose weight.

I lost 7 kg the first winter with the Antarctic Diet. I spent five to eight hours outside in the cold every week, going for walks or doing photography. I generally walked an average speed and after about half an hour my muscles were producing enough heat that I could take off my gloves or unzip my jacket. I was only hungry on occasion, since constant hunger is one of the main reasons people quit their diets. I limited my consumption of wine and beer slightly, but otherwise, there were no forbidden foods. Of course, a single record does not make for a rule of thumb. Perhaps you will gain less weight or perhaps even more weight than I did. If you happen to be reading these lines on a cold winter day, close the book, bundle up and go out into the cold – but do not stop to check what your 745 Internet friends are up to before you do!